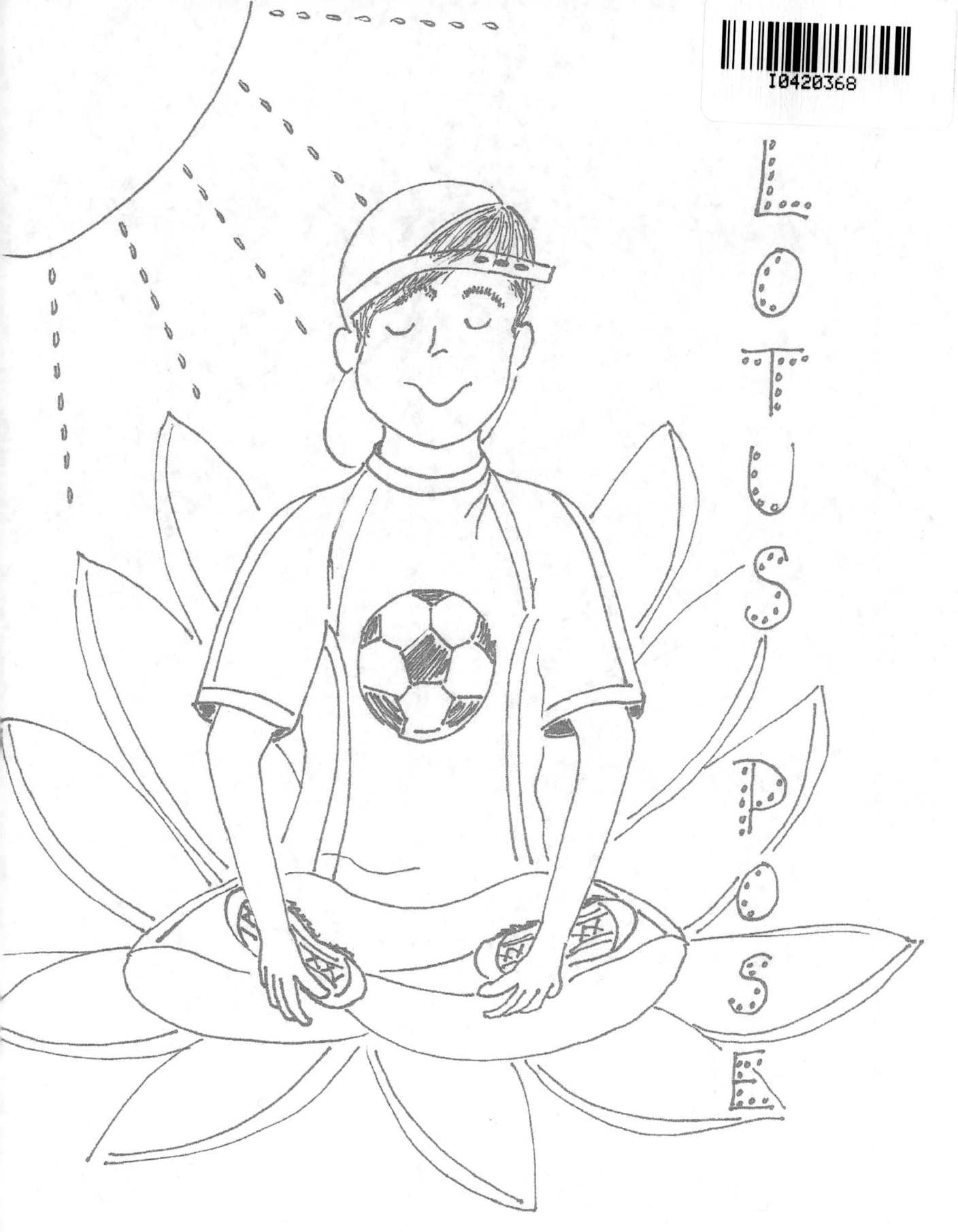

LOTUS POSE

HERE COMES THE SUN YOGA

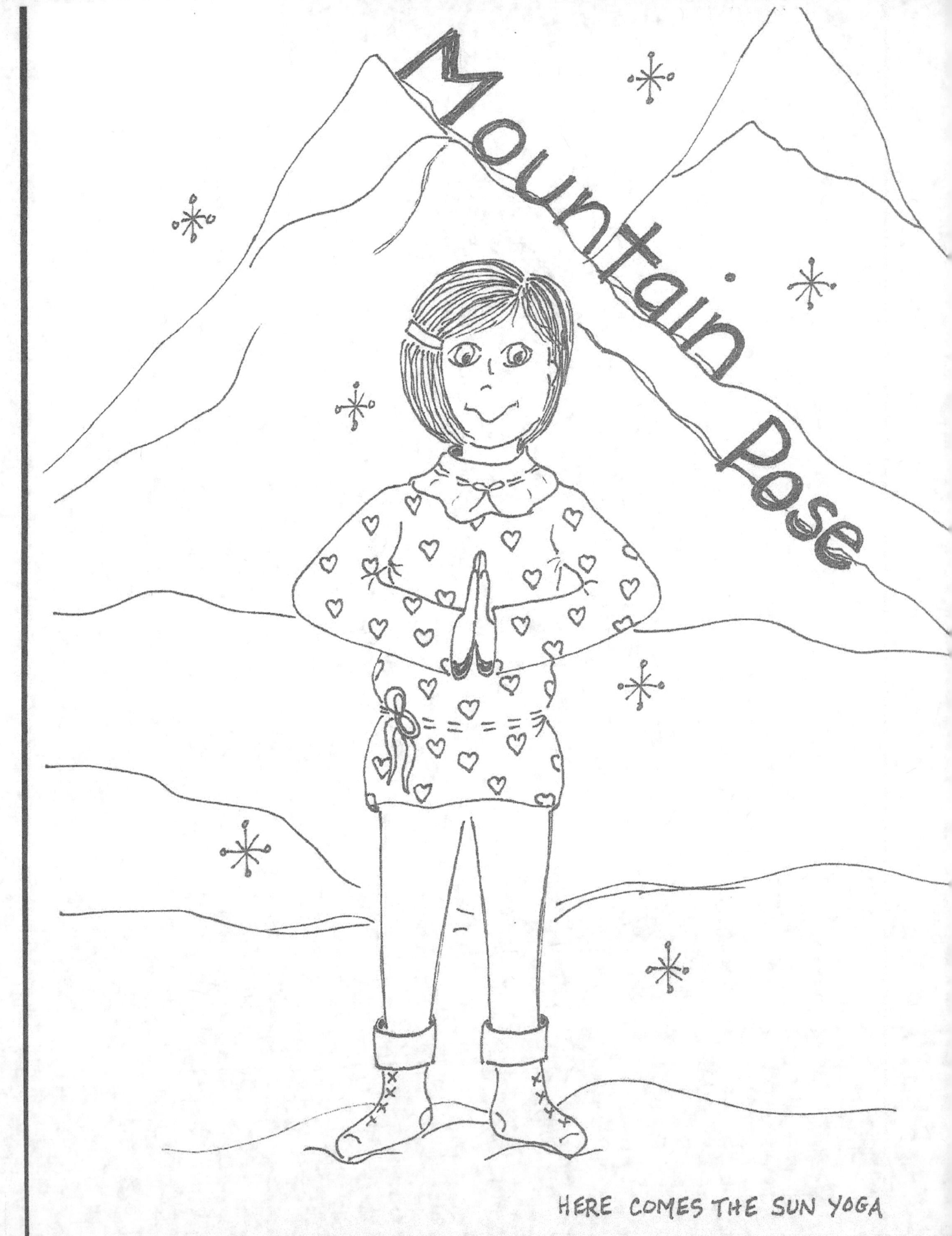

HERE COMES THE SUN YOGA

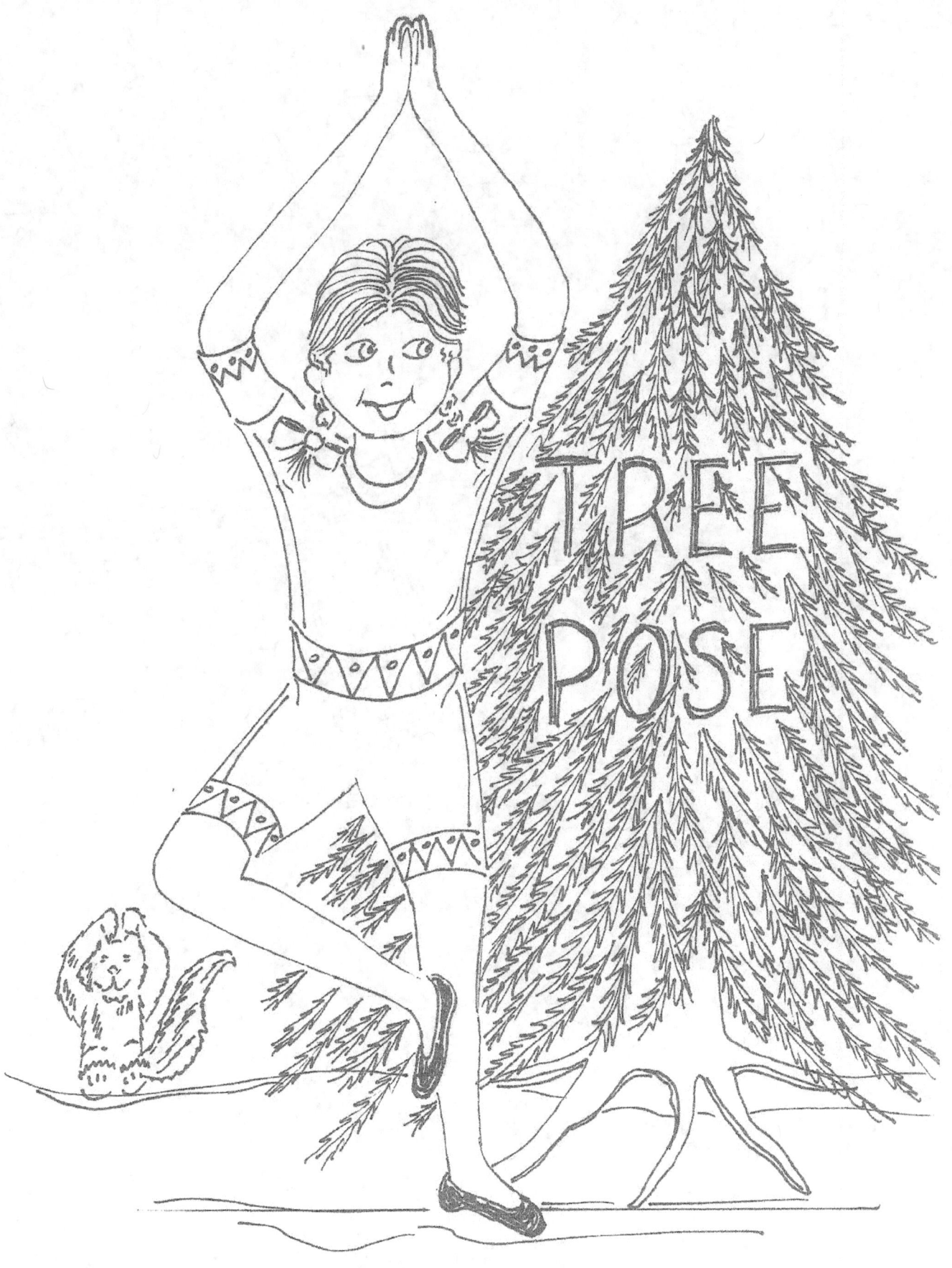

HERE COMES THE SUN YOGA

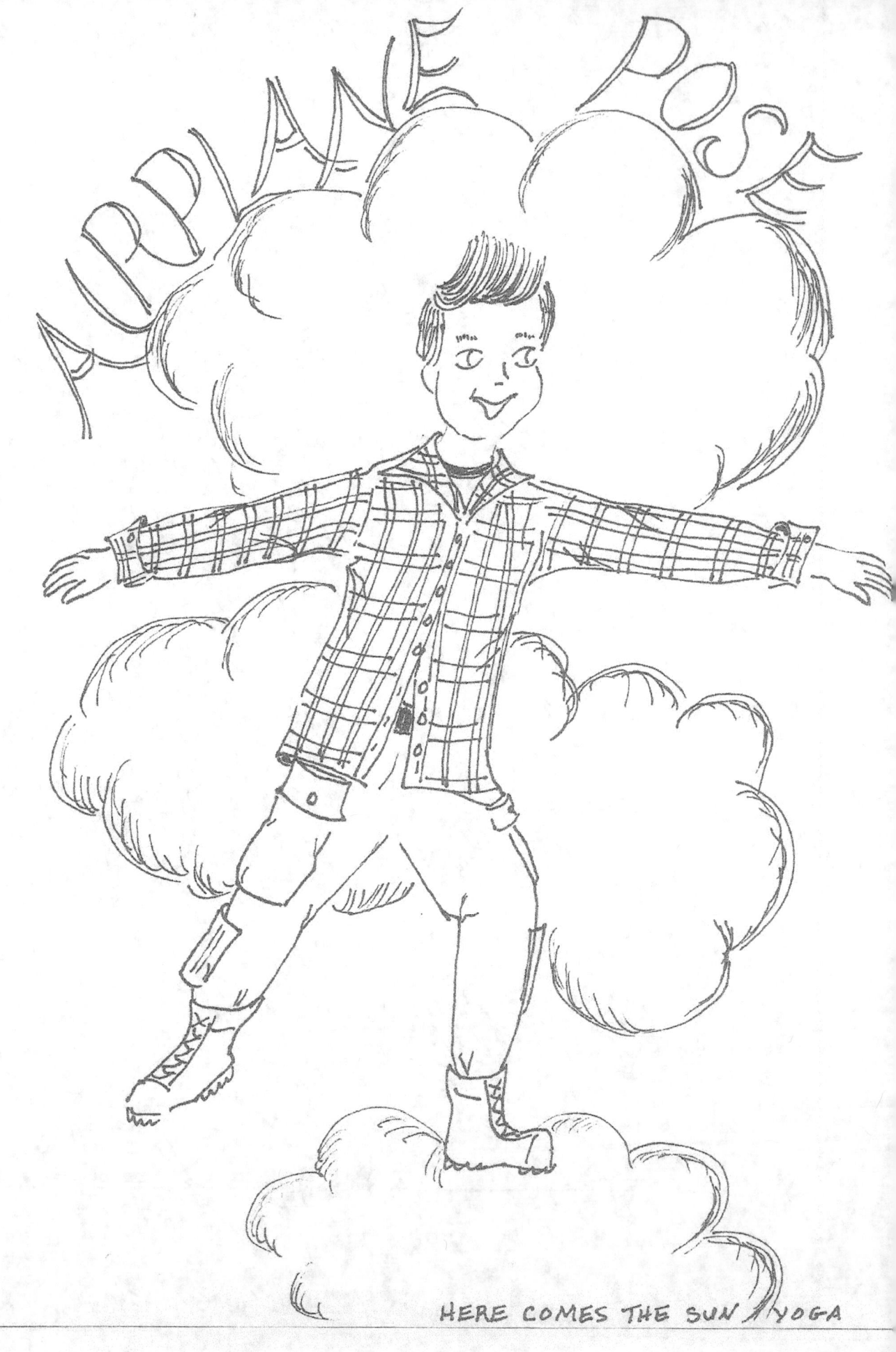

AIRPLANE POSE

HERE COMES THE SUN / YOGA

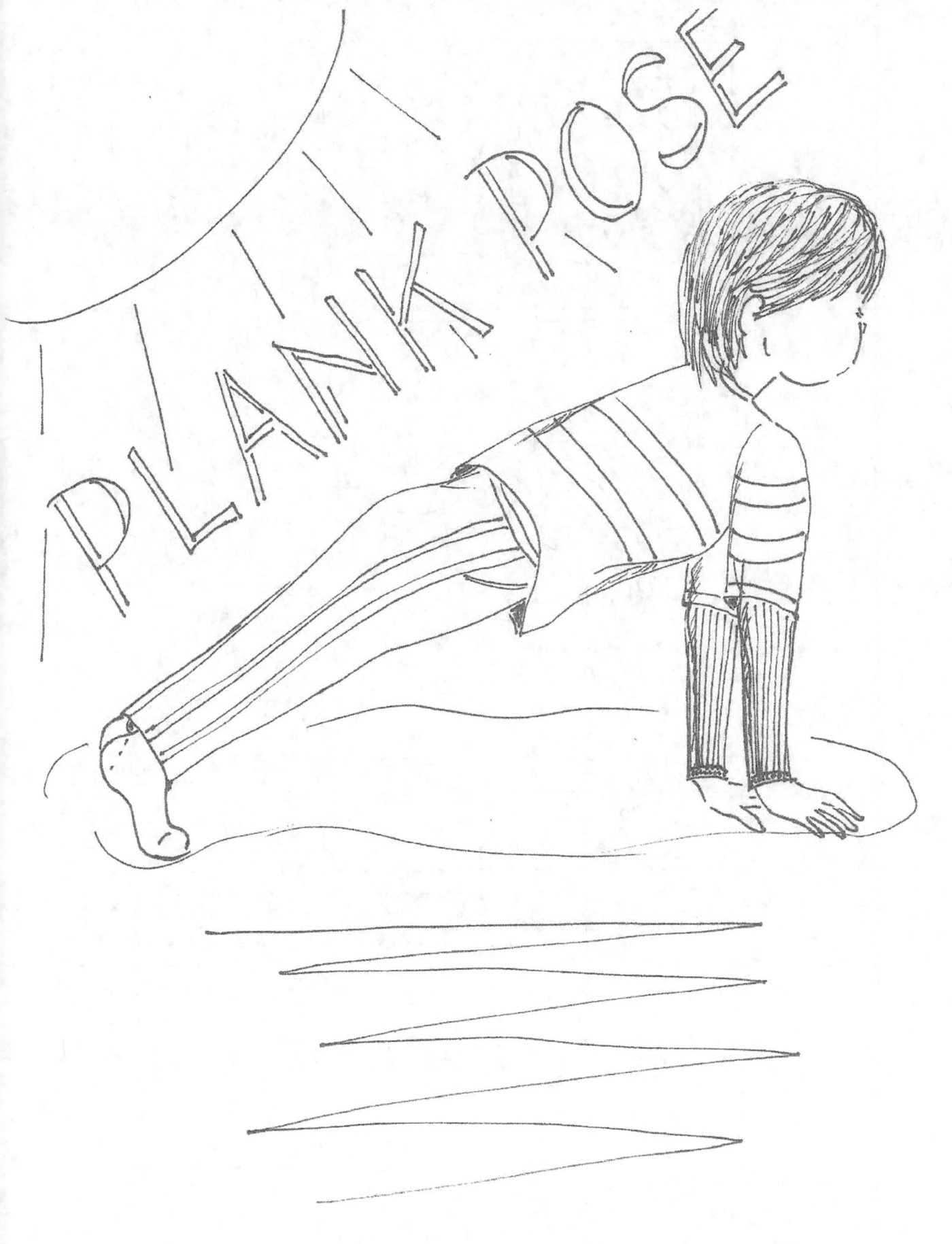

HERE COMES THE SUN YOGA

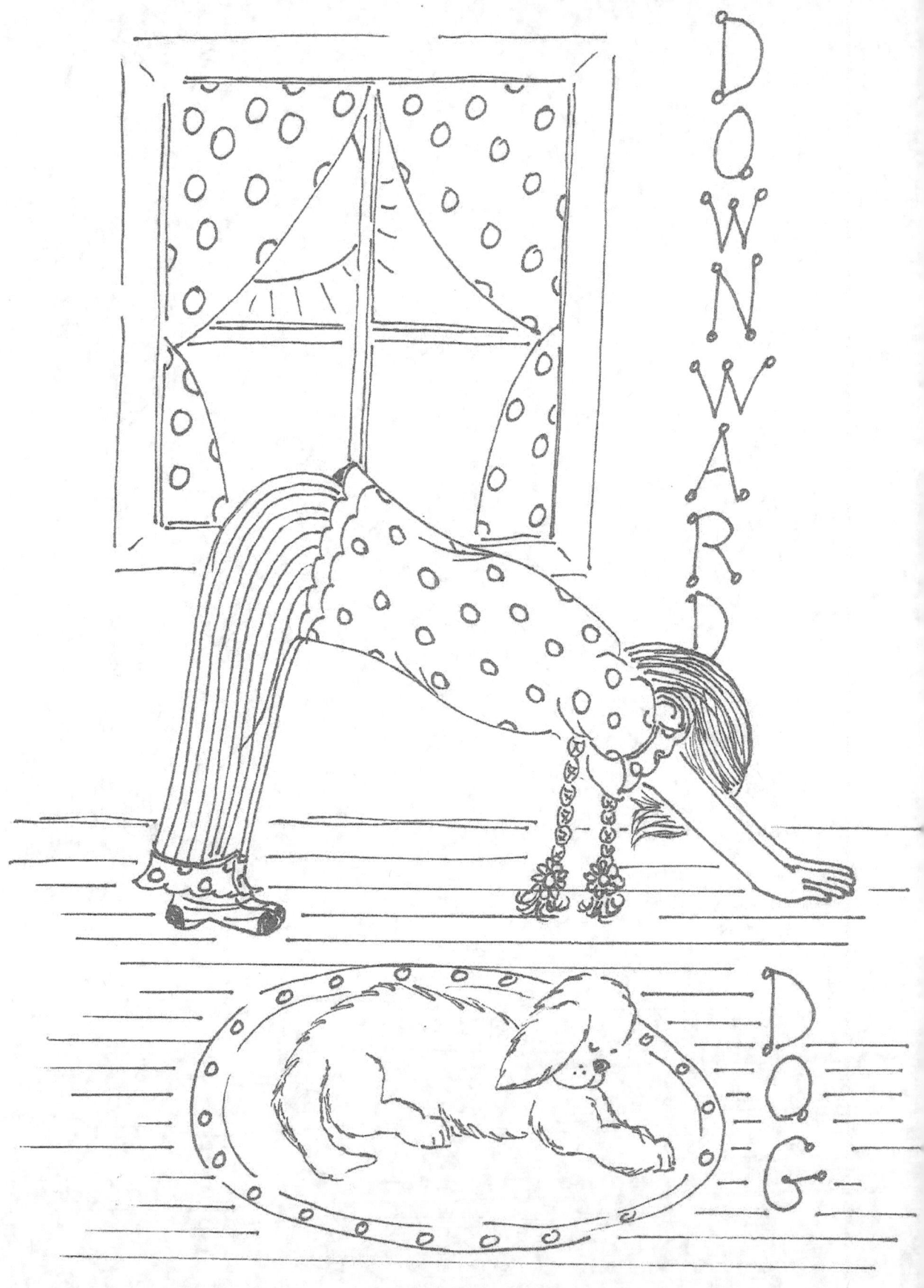

DOWNWARD

DOG

HERE COMES THE SUN YOGA

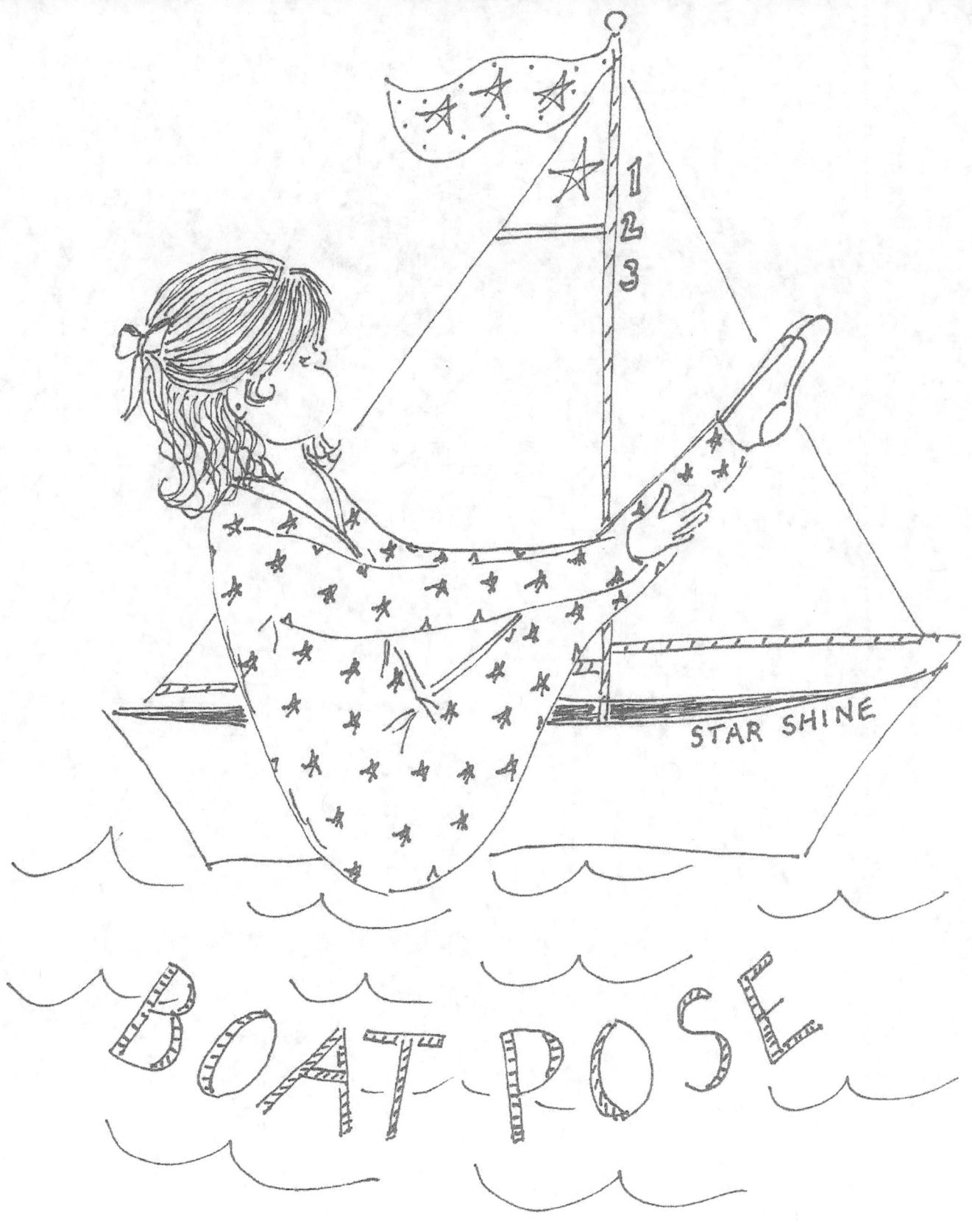

BOAT POSE

STAR SHINE

1
2
3

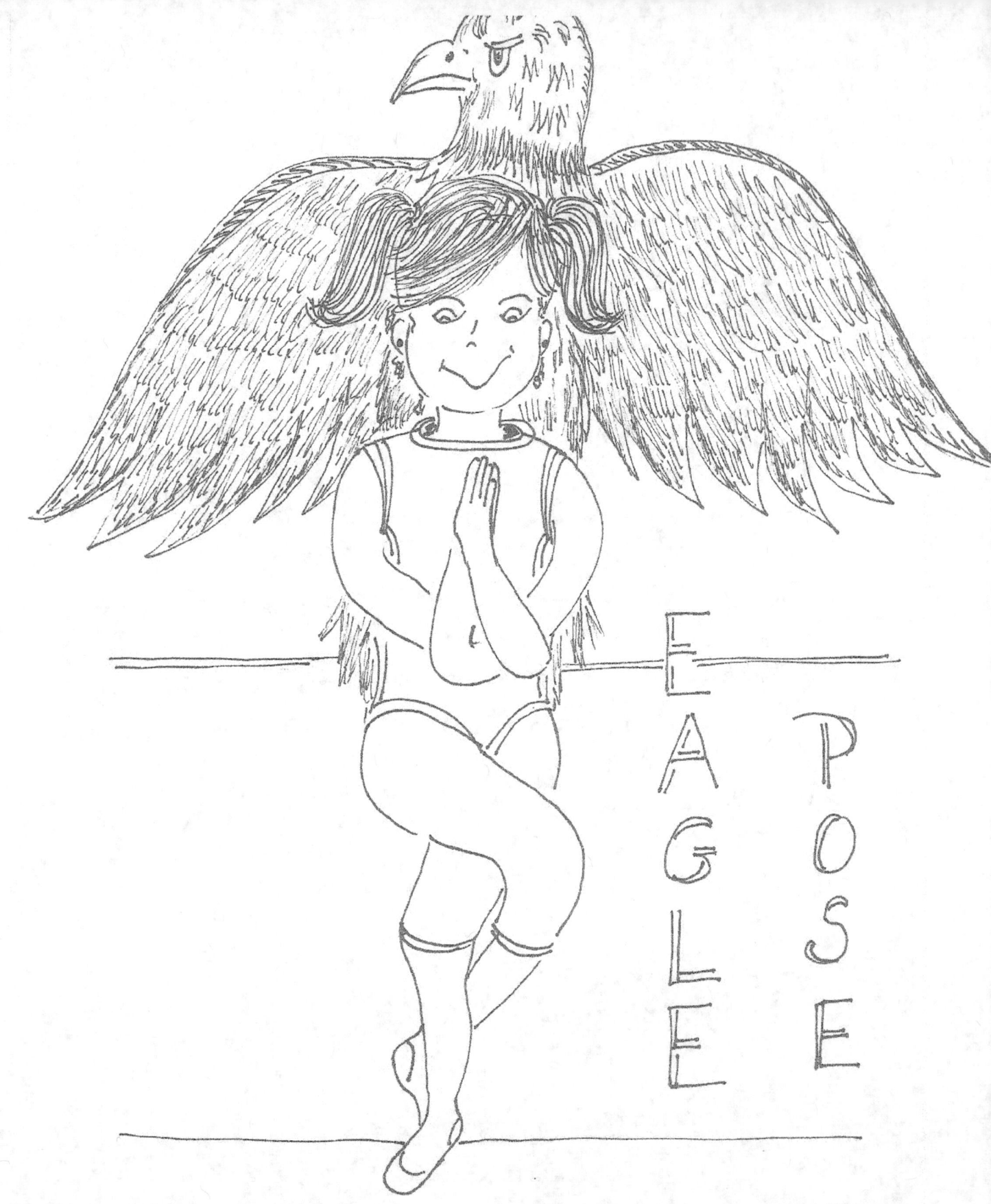

EAGLE POSE

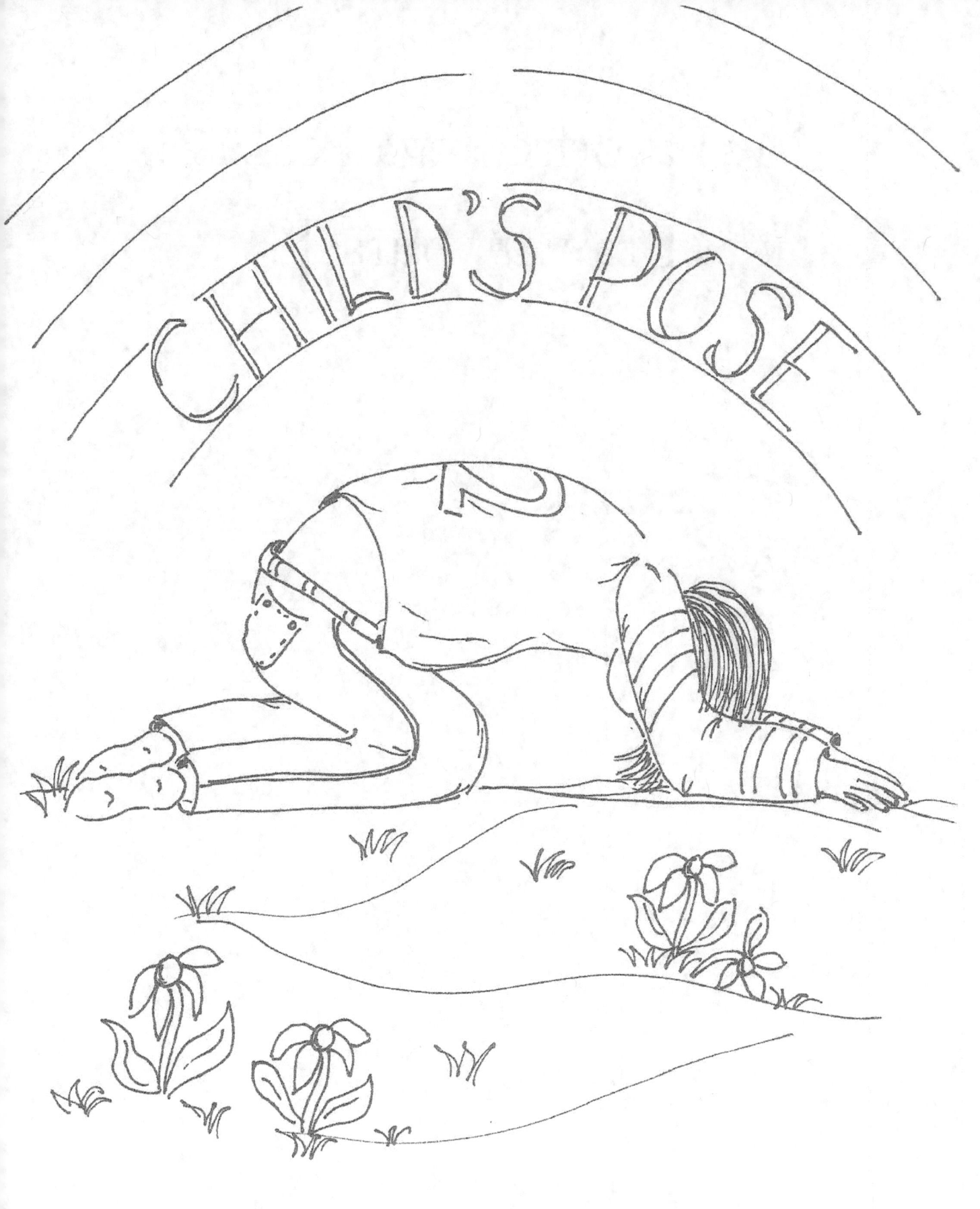

CHILD'S POSE

My Favorite Yoga Pose is....
Draw it yourself!

My Favorite Yoga Pose is....
Draw it yourself!

My Favorite Yoga Pose is....

Draw it yourself!

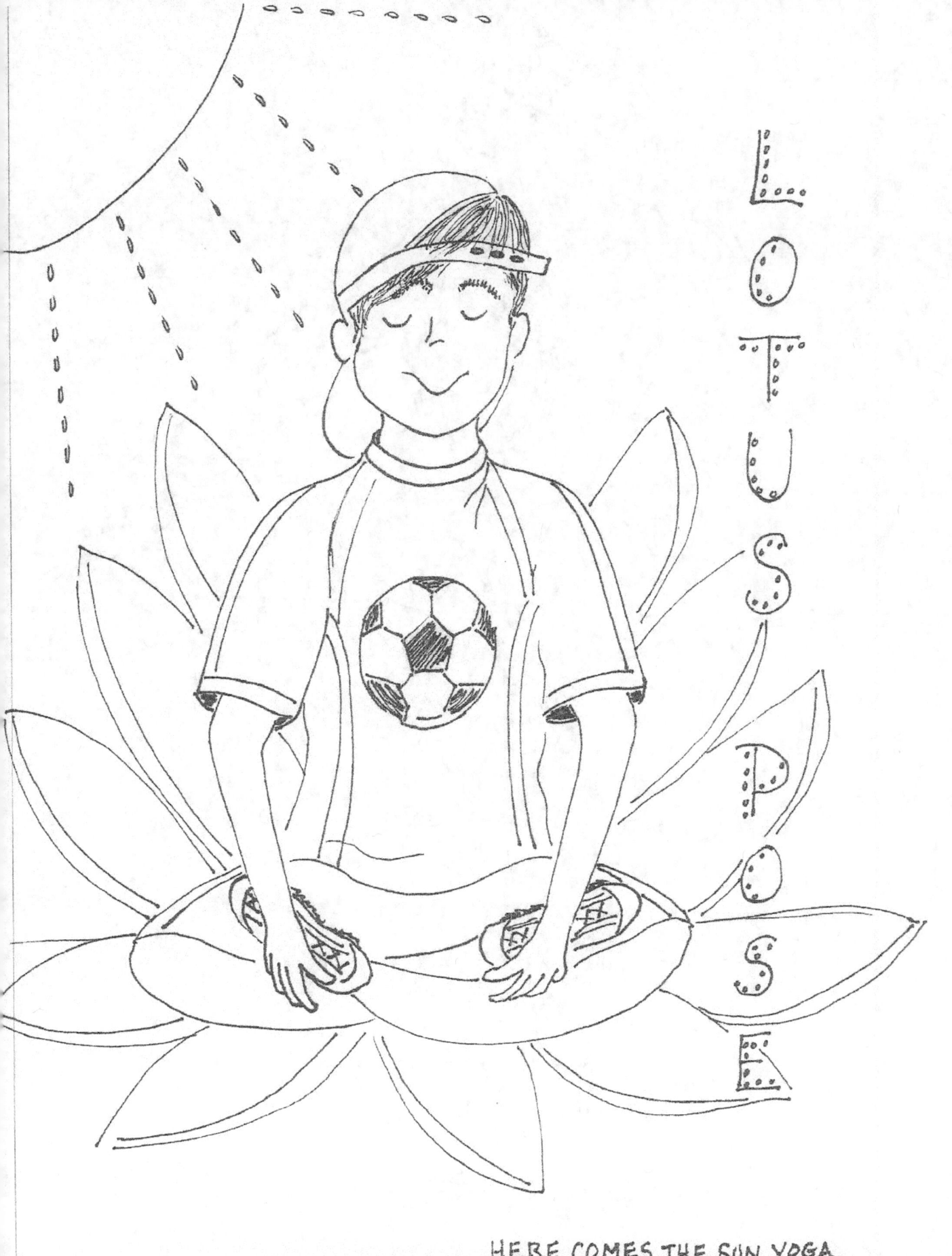

LOTUS POSE

HERE COMES THE SUN YOGA

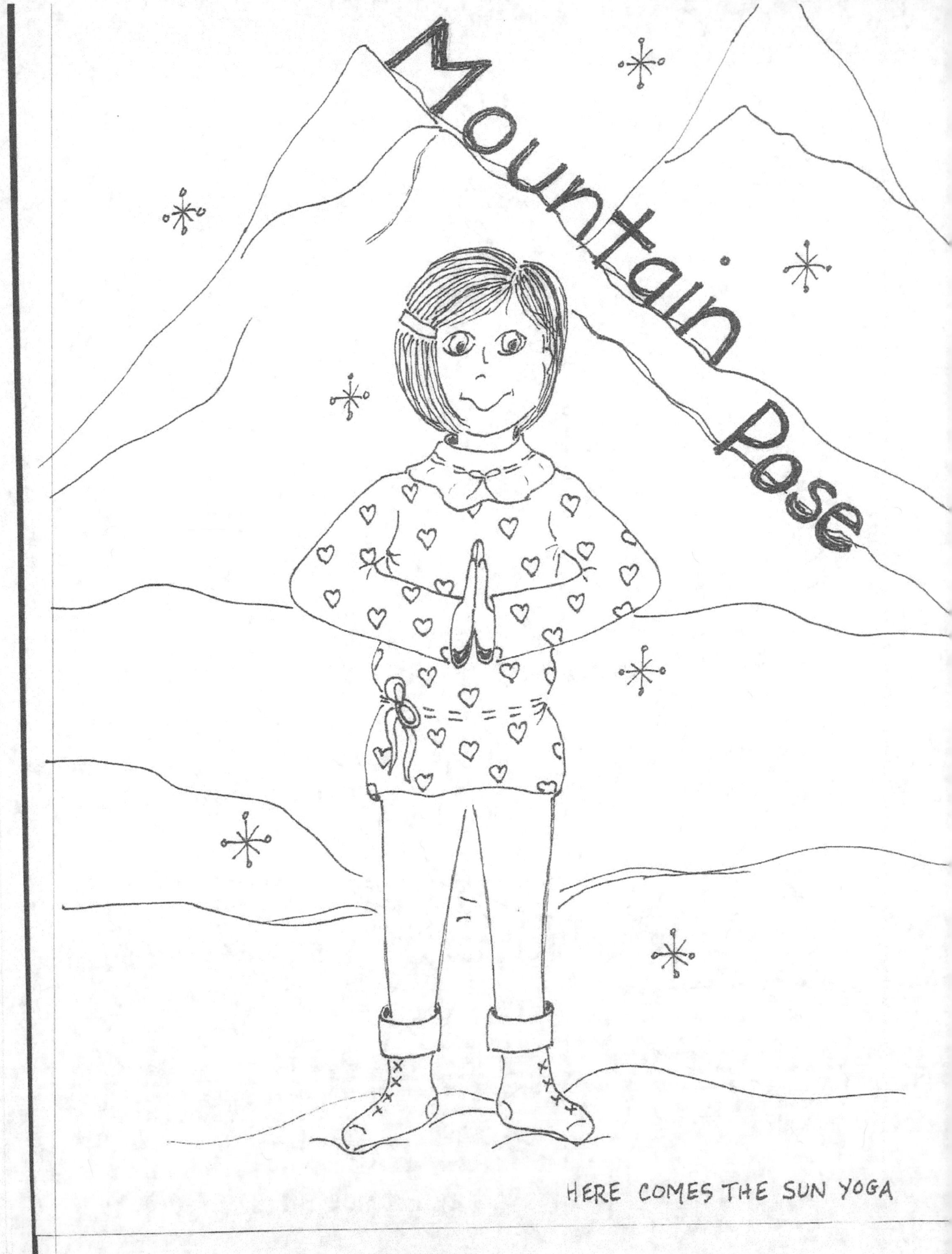

Mountain Pose

HERE COMES THE SUN YOGA

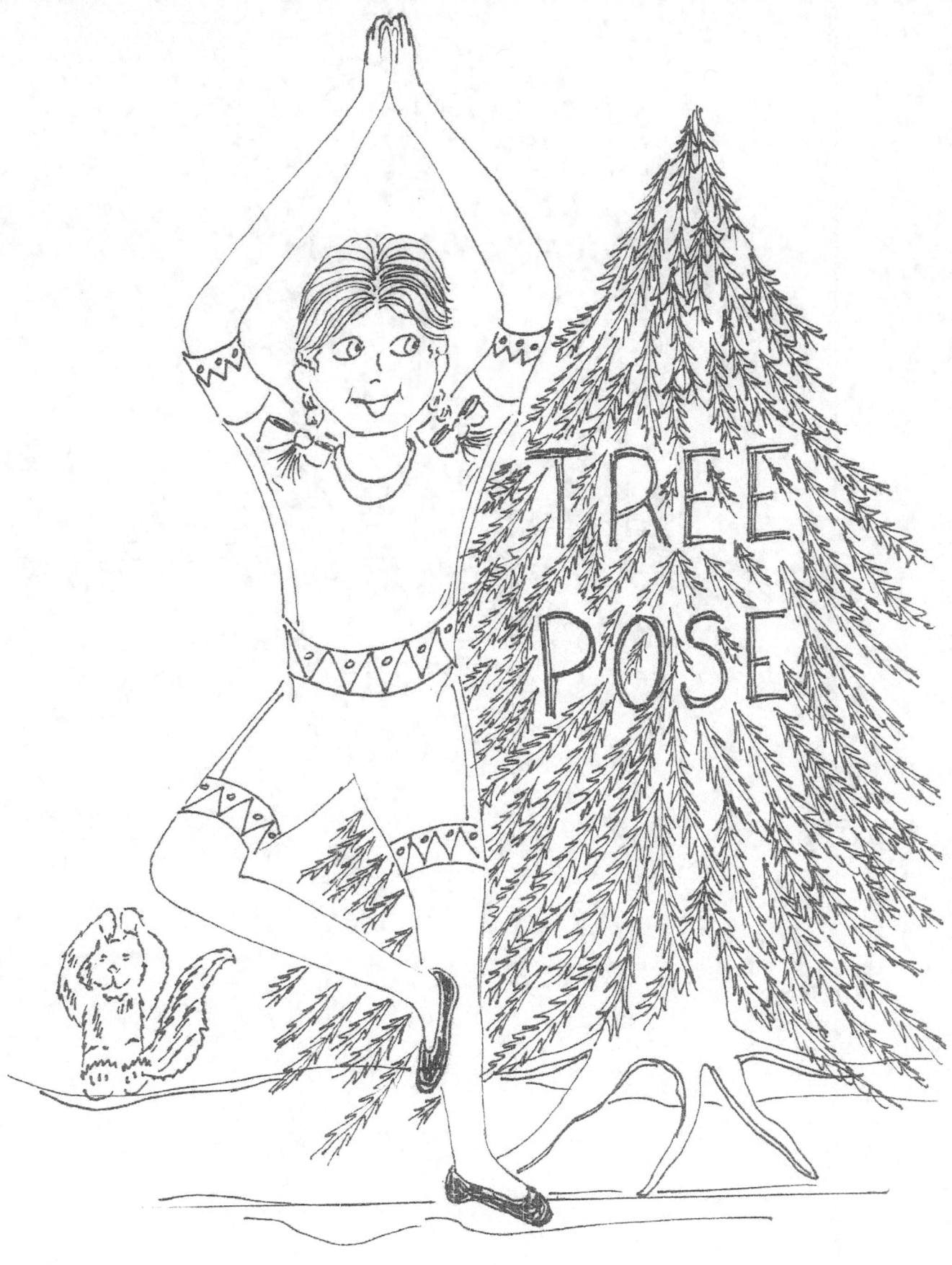

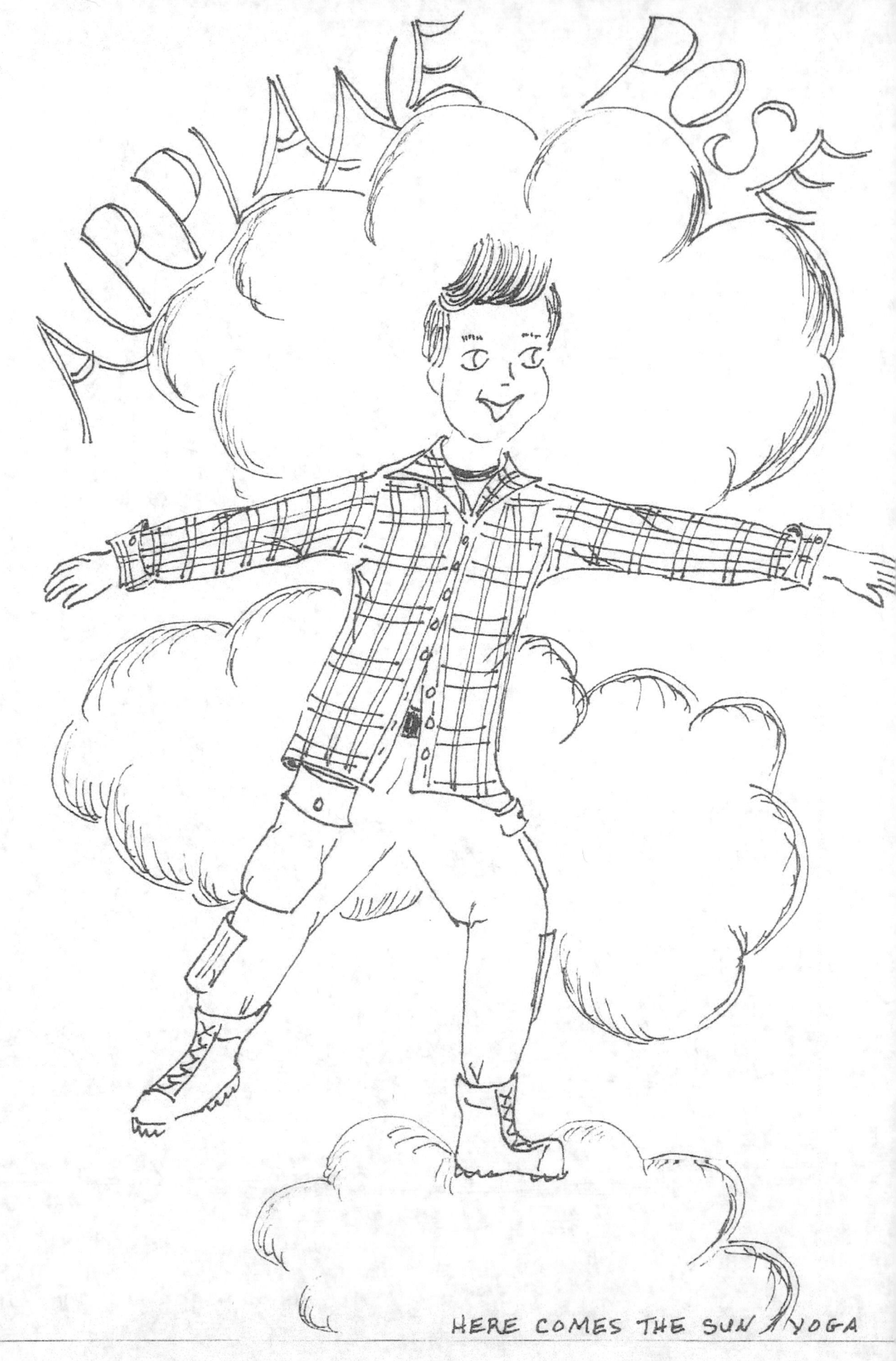

HERE COMES THE SUN / YOGA

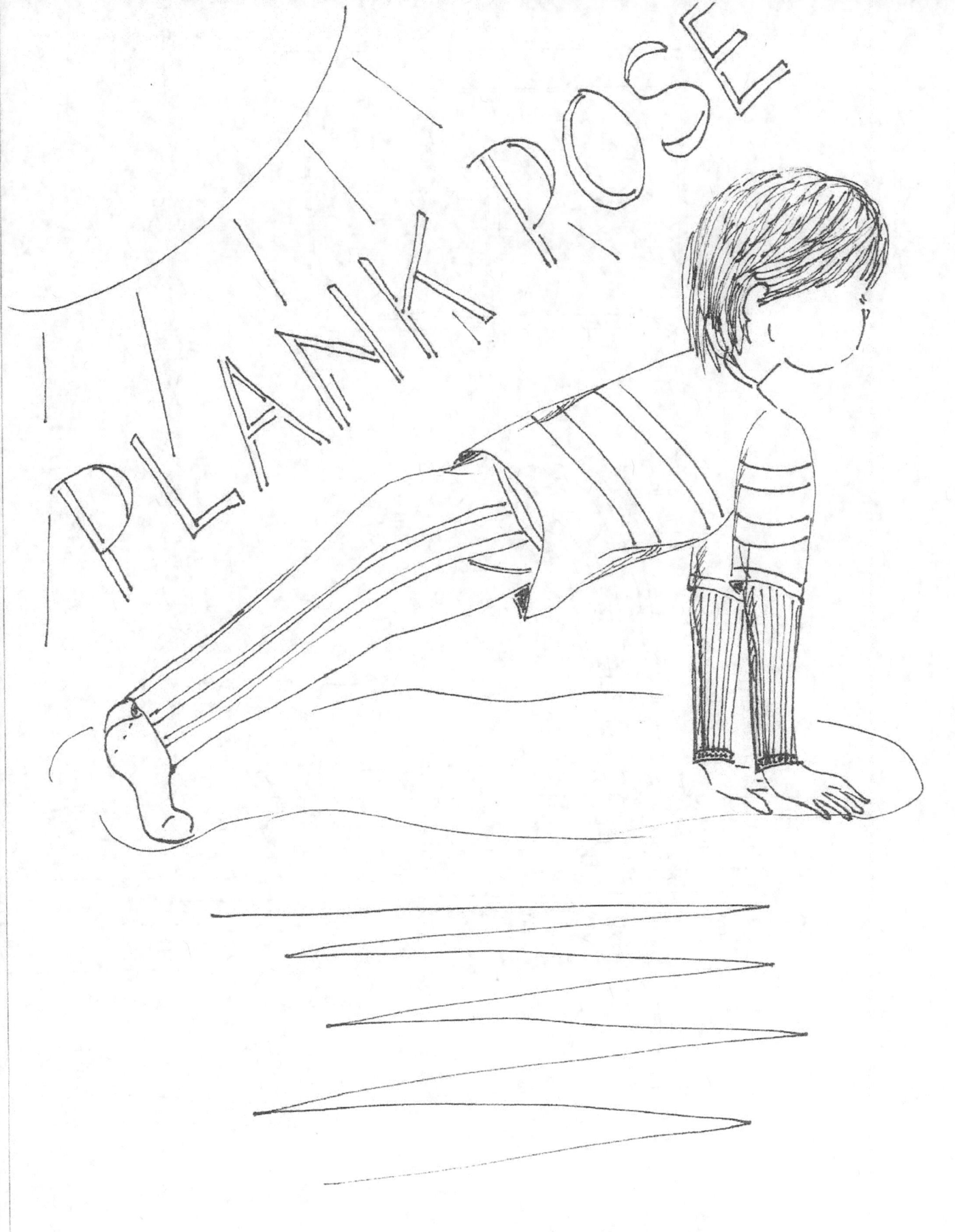

HERE COMES THE SUN YOGA

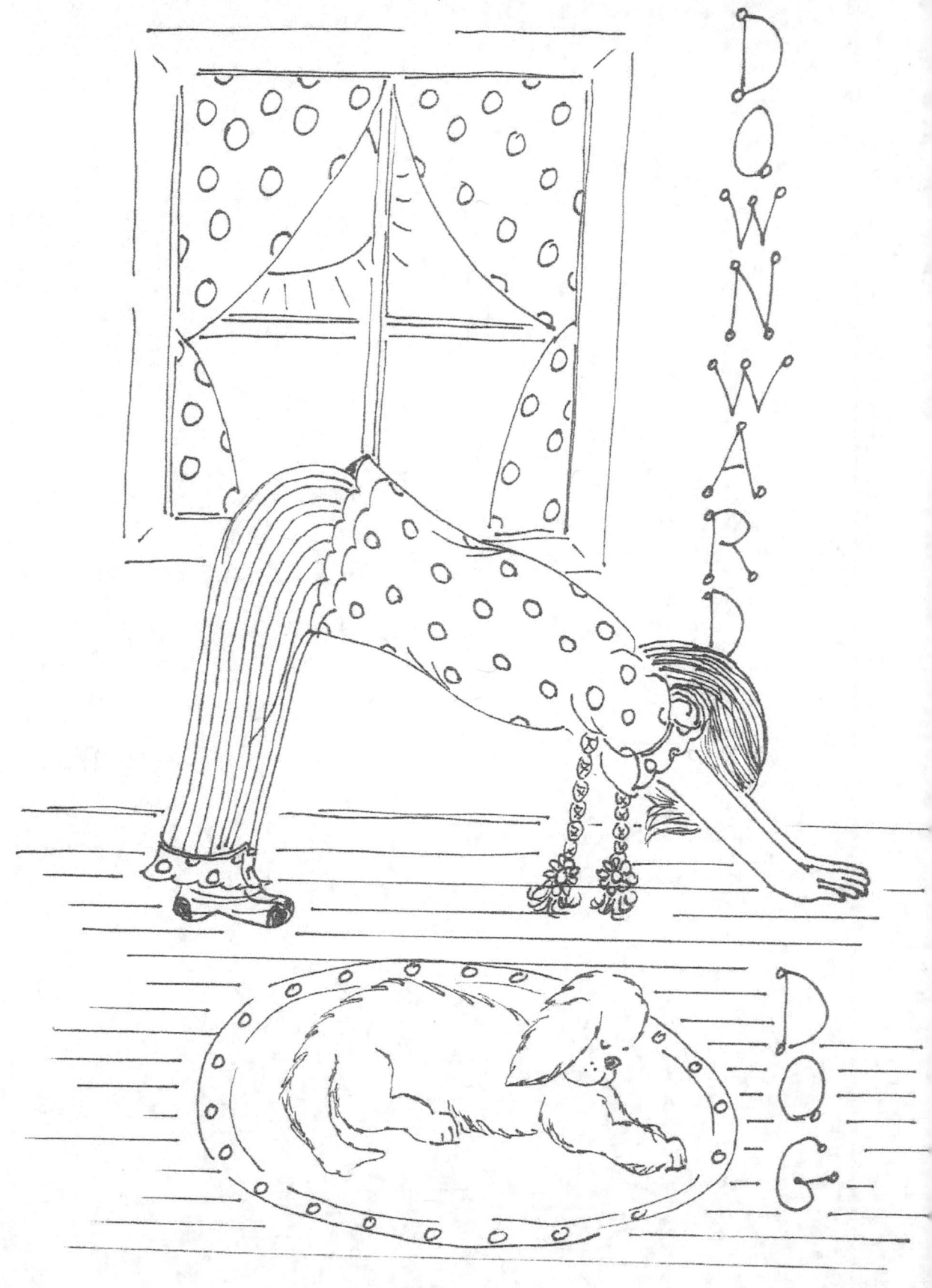

DOWNWARD

DOG

HERE COMES THE SUN YOGA

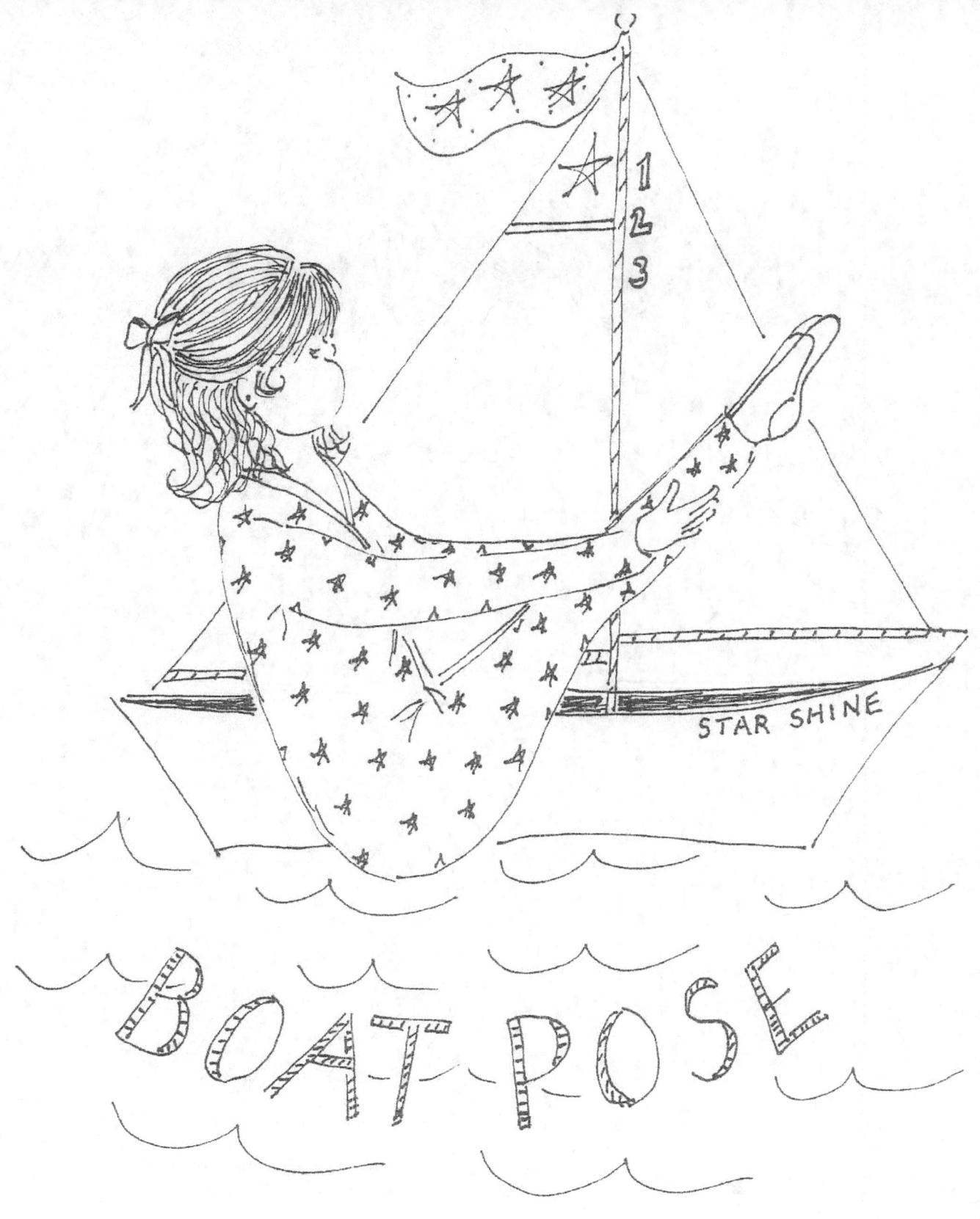

BOAT POSE

STAR SHINE

1
2
3

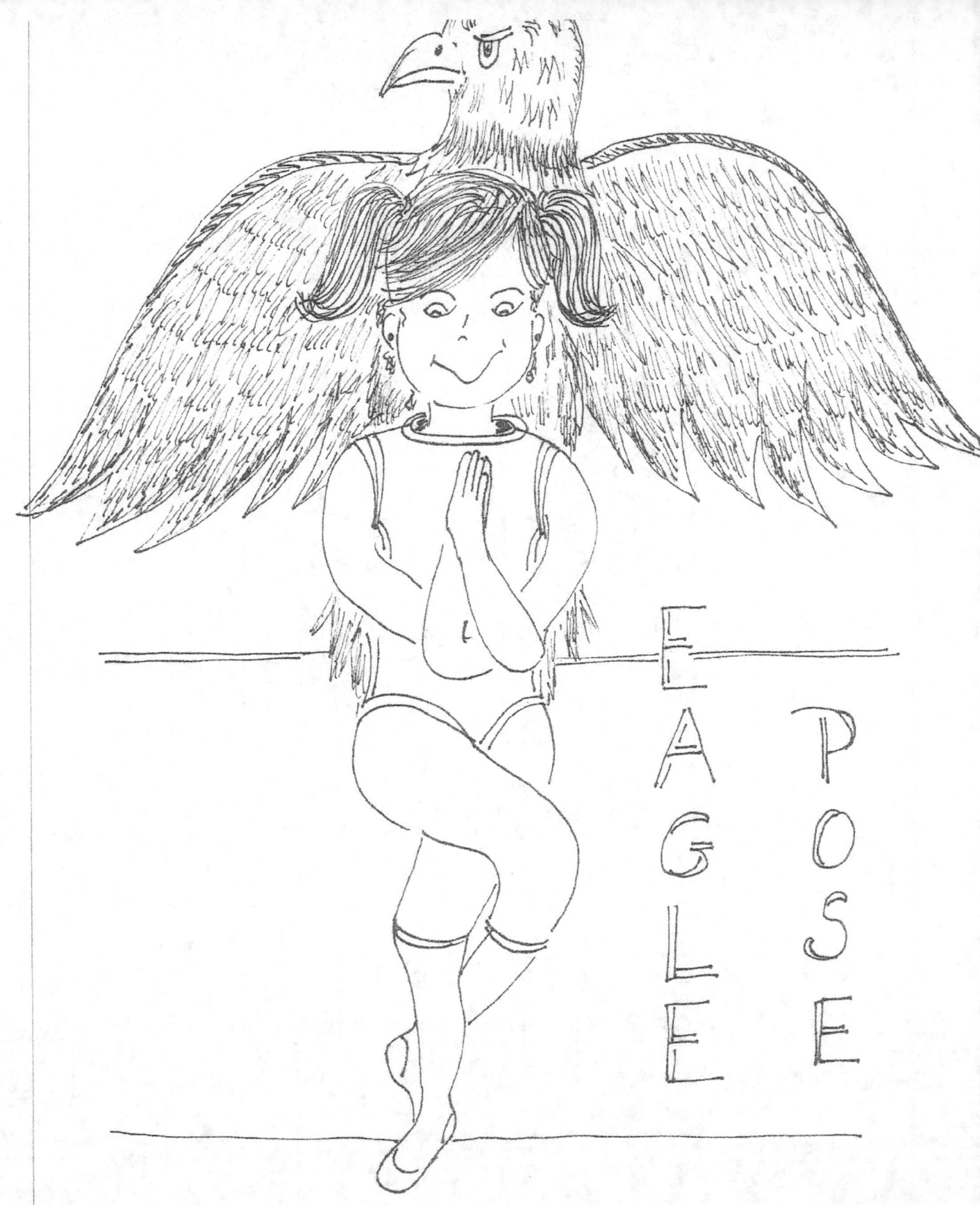

EAGLE POSE

HERE COMES THE SUN YOGA

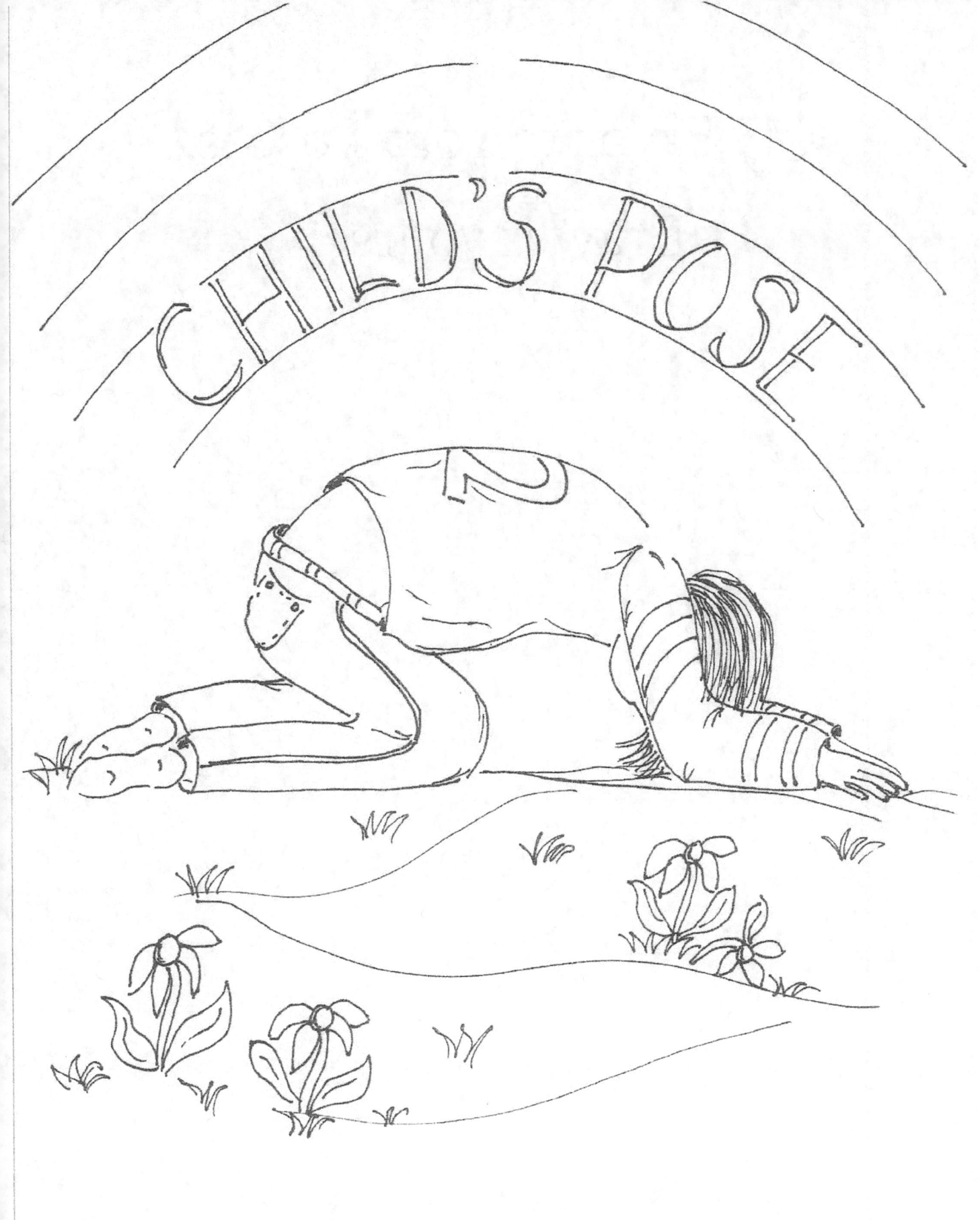

HERE COMES THE SUN YOGA

My Favorite Yoga Pose is....
Draw it yourself!

My Favorite Yoga Pose is....
Draw it yourself!

My Favorite Yoga Pose is....
Draw it yourself!

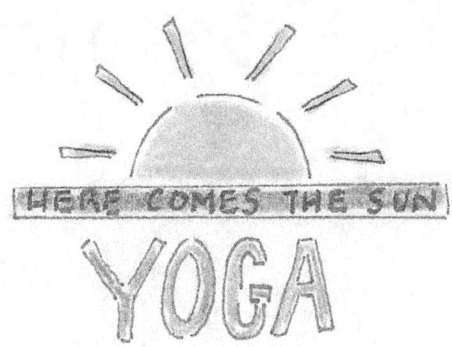

HERE COMES THE SUN
YOGA

Sharon Marrama
WWW.HERECOMESTHESUN.COM

TIME TO COLOR
8 .7. 6. 5. 4
Coloring Books

Patricia Hillenbach
phillenbach@gmail.com

∽ 2015 ∽

www.ingramcontent.com/pod-product-compliance
Lightning Source LLC
Chambersburg PA
CBHW081144280526

45787CB00007B/3216